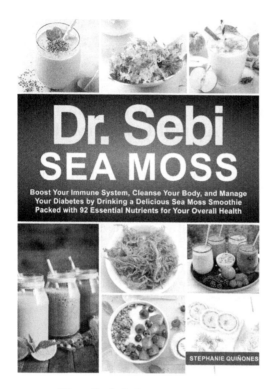

Dr.Sebi Sea Moss

Boost Your Immune System, Cleanse Your Body, and Manage Your Diabetes by Drinking a Delicious Sea Moss Smoothie Packed with 92 Essential Nutrients for Your Overall Health

Ebook ASIN: B08R12HYN1
Paperback ISBN: 9798568571360

Dedication

I would like to dedicate this book to Dr. Sebi for sharing the knowledge of the power of Alkaline, Electric Food, and the Medicinal Herbs diet that heals the body and cures diseases. You have inspired me to change my nutrition in my life and make life so much satisfying to live.

I honored your hardwork and determination in providing us with the knowledge to overcome adversity. I will not take this for granted and will pass along your powerful knowledge about health and nutrition through the Alkaline and Electric Foods diet.

Table of Contents

Introduction

Health and wellness are always a great thing, and there is a lot that you can do to achieve it. However, there is one health fad that many people have grown curious about. That is sea moss.

Sea moss may seem a bit strange. But, this naturally-occurring entity has many different health and wellness benefits, that you may not even be known. In this book, we'll tell you a bit more about sea moss, what it is, and the benefits of such.

This naturally-occurring moss however is one which shouldn't be discounted. In our world, it's seen as a superfood, but for some, it is considered almost miraculous. And the amazing thing is, it's readily available too! That's right, you can use sea moss. You might've heard about this from celebrities, and while some regard it as "trendy" there are real properties that are there, and we'll go into the true benefits, some of the amazing vitamins and minerals which are present in this, and of course, anything else that you may need to know about sea moss.

We'll also go into the different ways you can use it, and some cautions that may come with this as well. If you're curious about this, read on, and find out a bit more about sea moss, and what it can do for you.

Chapter 1

So What is Sea Moss?

Sea moss is actually great for a lot of things. While seaweed has always been regarded as a superfood, sea moss not so much. But, sea moss does have its own sort of benefits to it too, and we'll go over exactly what it is in this chapter, and in a general sense what it can do for you.

What is Sea Moss?

Sea moss is usually called Irish sea moss or Irish moss. There are some variants, but in a lot of cases, it's a seagrass, which essentially is a patch of plant life, typically on rocks and the ground, and it flourishes due to contents not only in the water, but in the environment around them, and it helps with growth as well.

This is a red seaweed that grows in inlets and tidepools all year around.

It's harvested in New England commonly, in order to extract what's called carrageenan, which is a carbohydrate that's gelatinous and it's commonly used in cosmetics and baked goods.

So yes, chances are you've probably had this before in some way, shape or form.

But sea moss also can be eaten by itself, and is used in stews and soups. This is definitely a fun little superfood, and it does have some great benefits.

So why did it become popular? Well, we can thank Kim Kardashian for that one.

Seeing Kim sipping on a sea moss smoothie has attracted attention by many people, and the healthy eating lexicon has since then burst into curiosity about this superfood. Why this? What's so special about it?

This red algae actually has an interesting history, and while it may seem strange that sea moss is popular, it certainly has a reasoning for it.

Well, we'll go into the benefits of this as well, but many proponents like it for its numerous benefits.

The History

The history of Irish moss is actually quite interesting.

Typically, this moss is found around the Atlantic coast. While commonly found in the US, it's actually also seen in Ireland and parts of Europe.

The moss got its name because during the potato famine in the 1800s, this was actually something that they ate. During the potato famine, they consumed this in order to get the nutrients needed, and since then, the name "Irish" stuck around with it.

There is also Jamaican sea moss, since this is also typically found around the coasts there too.

This is also called the carrageen sea moss due to that ingredient, since it's an additive along with a means to thicken different recipes.

It actually goes even further back too.

This algae has been in our diet for a millennia. While it has been found mostly in Ireland and the Caribbean, it's also been used in other cultures for many years, and is seen as a tonic to help with various problems on a general spectrum.

Where is it Found?

Typically, this is found on the rocks along the coastlines of the Atlantic. It is a red algae that's been taken out of the water, and it is stored in the fridge in many cultures.

How to Get it?

Typically you can get it in four forms, and they are:

1. A gel
2. Bath powder
3. Pill
4. Foods you consume

There is a difference in each form though, and we'll go over a few of the differences here.

Are the Gel, Bath Powder, and Pill the Same?

The sea moss gel that you see is actually sea moss that's put in spring water and soaked. This is done to help get rid of the extra salt and iodine, and from there, this is blended together in order to create a gel form.

Sea moss capsules are essentially the powdered form of sea moss, but stored on vegetarian capsules, so pretty much like many other nutritional supplements that you may have as well.

The powder form is essentially sea moss which has been dried and then crushed into a powder form, and from there, you can typically put it in a drink to add the sea moss supplement to it.

This is also how the food version is typically done, since in many cases you can simply infuse the sea moss directly into it.

Is there a big difference between these though? No, there isn't. they're the same thing, with the same great and amazing nutrients that are in there. For many people, they like to use one, or the other, or sometimes a mix of both.

It's totally okay to use either or, and it should be encouraged to use different kinds of means for sea moss, since they're great and wonderful means to get the nutrients that you love.

Man-Made Sea Moss: The Real Caution

Man-made sea moss is becoming more and more common when it comes to sea moss.

This is processed sea moss, and the problem is that this actually can alter the nutritional content within this.

According to Dr. Sebi, this type of sea moss is grown in brine pools, and it's artificially done.

These mass producers will take this directly from the ocean, attempting to replicate the same factors that are present in the ocean, but it isn't fully replicated.

With man-made sea moss, it doesn't have the properties that the ocean has, and in many cases, it actually can affect the quality. In the ocean, the sea moss is not only getting nutrients from the ocean water itself but also the air, the sun, and even the rocks that it does grow upon. The salt and other nutrients that are in ocean water also affect this.

Man-made sea moss tends to be much saltier, and it doesn't have the same components that regular sea moss tends to have, and this affects the quality of it. Typically, it is about three times the size, and has a lot more mucilage than other sea moss from the ocean itself.

So you aren't getting as much quality nutrients from this. You should make sure to avoid pool-grown from farms as well.

Difference Between Real and Man-Made Sea Moss

You may wonder if there is a way to tell the difference between this. Well, besides the nutritional content and the mucilage, typically those that are grown in a brine pool tend to have a much lighter color than those natural types of sea moss, and it typically has a much saltier taste.

It also won't have as many other minerals, so you're getting the salt content, and it can be almost too much, but not enough of the other nutrients.

And of course, this can affect the quality of the sea moss and how it affects you too.

There are four ways to tell the difference between real and fake.

First, you can tell by the look. This is obvious, but real sea moss is not grown evenly, and real sea moss may have some more thickness to it than others. Whereas the fake sea moss looks perfect—almost too perfect!

Next is the salt grains. Sea moss soaks up the water that it's in, so you'll typically see these only on the surface of the water, and it typically won't have as salty of a taste. On the flip side, if your sea moss looks like powdered sugar dusting, that's a sign you may have something fake on your hands.

Then there is the other seaweed that's in it. Real sea moss may have some other seaweed in it. That's because sometimes other seaweed comes along as a straggler. Not necessarily a huge problem, but it's there. In tanks and pools, you literally just see the sea moss, and it looks only like that, and typically has a dirtier look to it.

Finally, there is a difference in tone and color. With real sea moss, you typically have some variants of color, but they're slight. It's there. However, if you have sea moss that's all there looking the same and looks too even and perfect, chances are that's some fake sea moss on your hands. If you notice that there isn't much variation, it typically is processed, so you should make sure that you don't buy that.

Sea moss is great, but you never want to buy the same variations of this, but instead, get yourself something that's real, authentic, and actually is grown naturally, otherwise, you're missing out on the real nutritional value.

Now you know a little bit more about sea moss, let's explore all of the different kinds of sea moss you can get, and the benefits of such too.

Chapter 2

The Different Kinds of Sea Moss

Sea moss comes in a variety of different types. Let's go over the different kinds of sea moss you can get, what they entail, and the best jones for you to get.

Jamaican Sea Moss

Probably the most popular type next to Irish sea moss is Jamaican sea moss. This is typically sea moss, which is found along the Jamaican coastline, and is known for 92 different trace minerals within it that are vital for the human body to function correctly.

It's incredibly nutrient dense, and typically is made in a restorative gel or jelly, and is almost always tasteless and odorless, so it's easy to use in different dishes. It is typically the same as Irish moss, and they have virtually the same properties.

Chondrus Crsipus

This is what's commonly known as Irish moss, or carrageen moss in most cases, and this is grown along the Atlantic coast, usually in Europe or in North America.

This one typically has a color that goes from greenish-yellow to a reddish color or even a dark purple and a purplish brown as well.

Typically the primary component of this one is mucilaginous carrageenan, which is over half of its weight. It's also 10% protein and 15% dry weight mineral and also sulfur and iodine too in some cases.

Typically this can be boiled too, and it can grow up to 100 times of its weight within water alone.

This is probably the most popular type of sea moss out there and what most people are into as well.

Genus Gracillaria

This is typically referred to as normal sea moss in most cases, and is called "golden sea moss" in a lot of cases, since it has a golden color to it, compared to the reddish sea moss of the other kinds.

Some people say that this one is not "real" sea moss since it doesn't have the reddish color.

The reason why this one is a more golden color is because since they are closer to the sunlight, they typically get more light than red sea moss, hence why they are a more golden color too. With red sea moss, it's a lot darker, so it will be darker to absorb the light a bit more.

Typically, this is grown in the Java, Caribbean, and the Atlantic sea.

Eucheuma Cottonii

This is also similar to the Gracillaria types of sea moss. Typically, it's more of a lighter, golden color since it's typically closer to the water surface, and it's also normally flowing in the open currents. This type of sea moss is found in the same locations as the previous one, but it tends to be in clearer waters with more currents as well.

Compared to Chondrus Crispus, this is actually a lot rarer too, and typically grows a lot slower. This one is found in the color waters in the Atlantic Ocean, more towards the northern location, which is typically why it has a golden color, since it does require a bit more sunlight than most.

Other Kinds of Sea Moss

Really there are thousands of different kinds of sea moss in most cases.

They typically have the name algae rather than sea moss, and those, which include red algae and others, will most definitely be similar in nature to this.

There are thousands of types, and it can be varying in type.

Nori or purple laver is one that's typically found in Japan, Korea, and China for example. It's a thin, flat, and reddish-brown color that typically has a high level of production next to oysters in Japan. It is also eaten by the indigenous peoples in the Northwest in America and Hawaii, along with New Zealand and some British Isles.

Another is Aonori or otherwise known as green laver. This is a green seaweed very popular in japan, and typically it grows in deeper waters. It is a plant which is flat and leafy, and is only a singular cell thick, however, it's 20%% protein in size, and it has a high amount of vitamin and other content. Typically, rope nets are used to get this one out, and it is a singular generation of leafy plants.

Kombu is another one. This is a seaweed that comes from a species called Laminaria, and this is harvested along the northern part of Hokkaido, and about 10% of this is forming from the shores of Honshu as well. This is typically in a subtropical zone, and it is in calm waters. This is cultivated in a large part in China, Korea, and parts of Japan, and is about 10% protein, and 2% fat and has many useful vitamins and minerals.

Wakame is another one, and this grows along the rocky parts and bays of Japan, typically in the temperate zone, along with Korea and China. This is typically seen on the eefs and rocks in there, and it goes down to about 7 meters deep, and typically stops growing if the temperature in the water goes up above 25 degrees Celsius, so it is a cold water plant, and it has been found in France, Australia, and New Zealand. This one has a high dietary fiber content, and typically has a low level of fat content. This is a brownish-looking seaweed in many cases, and it's rich in vitamin B groups, including niacin as well.

Then we have Hiziki, which is a brown seaweed with a leaf structure that's finer than the others listed, and typically is found in the wild in Japan and Korea and in the sublittoral zones, and usually is processed in Korea and then given to japan. This is similar in nature to kombu, and typically most of the vitamins aren't present in this because of the processing that's done. The manganese and copper contents are very high, typically higher than kombu, and the fat content is low, but it has a lot fattier acid than the others do.

Finally, we've got Mozuku, which is a brown type of seaweed that's typically gotten from the southern islands of Japan, and typically only grows from October to April in the water. It's in more reef flats than in the water, and typically needs a more moderate current in order to get enough nutrients. This one typically has the salt removed in a lot of cases, and the salt is added and then removed, and it's exported to different areas.

Sea moss is a very generalized type of name, and while most of the time sea moss refers to red sea moss or regular sea moss, this does involve these variants too, and in many cases, it refers to the different types of plants that are out there.

The Best Types of Sea Moss

Really the best kind of sea moss is red sea moss, and regular sea moss.

Typically, golden sea moss is typically the one a lot of people like. This is Genus Gracilaria, and typically is found in a lot of warmer climates.

This one has a stronger look to it, and it does have a variety of red color to it. It's the most popular, and probably the best you can get quite easily, and readily as well.

Then there is red, or Irish sea moss. This is considered by some to be the "Rolls Royce" of sea mosses. This is typically one of the more popular forms of sea mosses, and a lot of people don't realize just how beneficial it is. It's a survival food, and is a superfood powerhouse now, and is considered some of the best out there.

It is a rarer sea moss, and typically isn't available all year around. However, this one has many amazing values. But, the one downside to this compared to golden sea moss, is that it can be costly. About half a pound can be at least 50 bucks. But, it is a great investment, especially if you love sea moss.

This one also has a lot of minerals within it, and while they're considered "essential minerals" that the body needs, some people do have some concern over the sheer amounts, but it definitely is a great idea if you're curious about sea moss.

Sea Moss Varieties

The main sea moss varieties are algae-types that are found on the rocks. Some do believe that seaweed does fall into these categories.

Whatever you choose to get though, sea moss has a lot of different properties that go along with this, and there are plenty of great benefits to be had with sea moss, and ones that you can use to your advantage too.

Chapter 3

The High-Immune Boosting Minerals of Sea Moss, and Their Benefits

Sea moss has a ton of nutrients in their profile. There are 92 of 102 different nutrients with them, and we'll list out a few of them here, and go into detail on some of the more important ones, and why they matter in the grand scheme of things.

The top minerals found in sea moss include:

- Calcium
- Folate
- Zinc
- Iron
- Sodium
- Copper
- Soluble potash
- Iodine
- Manganese
- Boron
- Magnesium
- Potassium
- Sulfur
- Phosphoric acid
- Selenium
- Alginic acid
- Laminarin
- Mannitol
- Nitrogen
- Vitamins A-E, along with Vitamin K

That's a lot already, and that isn't even everything, but let's get into a bit more detail on some of the more specific minerals located in sea moss.

Magnesium

This is one of the most abundant minerals in the body, and typically is part of 3-000 different enzyme regulations in the body, creating different reactions within the body which includes protein synthesis, nerve and muscle function, blood sugar control and even regulation of blood pressure.

It's also needed for producing energy, glycolysis, and oxidative phosphorylation as well, and it contributes to the bone structure and development, along with the synthesis of DNA, RNA, and also some antioxidants. It does play a role in the transport of potassium and calcium ions across different membranes, which helps with impulse control, muscle contraction, and of course, heart rhythm.

Phosphorus

This is the second most prevalent mineral in the body, and it's part of every cell in the body, and typically is found in teeth and bones as well, and is actually a percentage of our weight too. It's incredibly important for forming teeth and bones, plays a role in how fats and carbs are used, and of course, is necessary for protein and growth, maintaining, and also fixing up the tissue and cells. It also makes up ATP, which is what's used for energy in our body.

It's great for kidney and muscle function, but also is important for nerve health, and even a normal heartbeat too.

Typically it's hard to be deficient in this, but it can cause calcium to form in the soft tissues and muscles, and it can lead to kidney disease in rare instances if there isn't enough.

Iron

Iron is another very important mineral in our body, that we need for a variety of different functions. Iron is a part of something bigger called hemoglobin, which is a protein that's carried throughout our body out of the lungs.

It's important for our bodies and it is used in our muscles to keep oxygen around, and it can also be used with other enzymes and proteins.

If you don't have enough iron, you will experience something called anemia, and typically can cause issues including fainting, fatigue, and other problems. It typically is rare for it to be too prevalent in the body, but in some cases, too much iron does occur.

Zinc

Zinc is a trace element that is needed for your immune system. It actually is what keeps you from getting disease and illness as well, and it's responsible for at least 100 different enzymes. It also works to help with many different functions in the body, from energy to immunity. Typically it's used for your immune response, and also for attacking cancer cells. If you don't have enough of this, it can suspect you of many different pathogens.

Zinc also is good for treating issues with bowel movements and diarrhea as well. It typically can help with this issue especially in children.

It's also not just good for healing the body, but also improving your learning process and memory too, since it regulates how the neurons communicate to one another, and affects how memories are kept and how we learn as well. So if you want to remember things better, consider taking zinc.

Finally, along with treating the common cold, it can actually help with healing wounds by keeping the skin structure and integrity there, so if you have chronic wounds or even ulcers, you can start to reverse this better and better through the use of zinc supplements.

Collagen

This is another very popular protein within the body, and it does offer skin structure, can help with blood clotting, and it's been used in many cases as a supplement and ingredient in many skincare and beauty products.

This protein though is actually one of the main building blocks of your body, responsible for the tendons, ligaments, and even your teeth, blood vessels and corneas too. Think of it almost like a "glue" that holds everything together, and it's actually responsible for a third of the protein composition of the body as well.

Basically, it helps support the structure of your body, your connective tissues, and your teeth, and even your eyes. As you get older, your body makes less of this, and soon, your skin will look less supple and firm as you get older. It also can cause the cartilage in the body to weaken too. So, if you want to keep this looking supple and firm, then you should definitely consider collagen, for it's something that can be beneficial to many people.

Spirulina

Another very popular nutrient in this is spirulina. It's actually why it may have a little bit of a greenish color, and it's one of the most popular, and one of the most popular supplements. There are many different studies done on this, and more and more information has been discovered about spirulina that can benefit you.

Spirulina is part of this because it can attach to sea moss, since it grows in water, sand is a cyanobacteria that's oftentimes responsible for the greenish-blue hue. It is popular, and a little bit goes a long way, but it contains a bunch of other nutrients too, including protein, Vitamin B1, B2, B3, copper, and iron as well, and a lot of decent amounts.

Spirulina also has some powerful antioxidant and anti-inflammatory characteristics of it, so if oxidative damage is what you're trying to avoid, then this is probably one of the best things for you to have. It has a wealth of different antioxidants, and it can protect against this, and it can help prevent inflammation and inflammatory disease from taking root.

Sea moss has a bit of this in there, so not only is it housing some amazing benefits in it itself, but it also contains some other amazing properties that you may not find anywhere else.

Iodine

Then there is iodine, which is very important for thyroid health and wellness. This is a vital component of this, and it actually makes some of these hormones that contain this there.

A little bit goes a long way with iodine, and once you consume a little bit, it can go straight to the bloodstream, and from there, to the thyroid gland.

Now the benefits are definitely on a much broader level. They benefit literally every organ within your body. It's responsible for energy usage, growth, metabolism, and even repairing the tissues as well. If you don't have enough of this, it can actually be seen in a variety of conditions. Low iodine can cause your thyroid to either be overactive, or underactive, which can cause weight gain, a lack of energy, trouble sleeping and concentration, feeling cold and constipated, and problems with menstruation and even blood sugar issues.

An overactive thyroid or hyperthyroidism can result in everything moving too fast, where you're struggling with sleeping, having issues with focus, not being able to put on weight, and again, issues with body temperature and regulation.

Iodine also prevents goiter as well, which is something that is a change to your thyroid levels. The thyroid stimulating hormone typically helps counteract low thyroid levels. This typically can stimulate the thyroid gland on its own, but it does cause it to become enlarged, so if you notice your thyroid being even bigger, that's a sign of goiter, and a sign of thyroid issues.

You don't need a ton of iodine in order to prevent this, but it's important to understand that a little bit goes a long way with this, and it's one of the most prevalent minerals in sea moss, and it can help provide regulation to the body.

Other Important Components

With sea moss, some of this may be questionable with how much you should have. For example, the amount of aluminum that's in it may not be right, and there may be too much to cause an overabundance of certain minerals.

But there are a few which are important, and we'll go over a couple of them here, and why they matter.

First, there is selenium, which is used in many different applications, from baby formula to multivitamins, but it also is one of the main components of a healthy thyroid, ince it converts one type of the thyroid hormone to another as needed in the body. It an change from under different conditions too depending on what it's exposed to.

Selenium is great because it can prevent oxidative stress in the body, reducing the mpact or risk of cancer, stroke, aging, and Alzheimer's, reducing the mental health ffects, including depression, reducing complications that are associated with Iashimoto's disease, improving the immune system, and also reducing asthma ymptoms in the body. This contains a lot of it, and it's important that you understand hese benefits too, since they are prevalent, and great for you as well.

The other major part of this is laminarin, which is something that's found only in lgae and seaweeds, and it's responsible for the storage of Glucan, a polysaccharide, and lays a big role in many medical properties.

This does have anti-inflammatory, antioxidant, antiproliferative, antiapoptosis, ntiviral, anticoagulant, antitumor, and immunostimulatory properties that go around vith this. This is typically done during photosynthesis, and it's important for the life ycle of many of these unicellular organisms. This is a carbohydrate for sea moss, and t's important. It is used in a lot of cases in phytoplankton as well, and this is actually a big part of many of the nutrients.

So as you can see, it's very important for a lot of people to have, since sea moss ontains so many different properties.

A lot of people are worried about sea moss because there is still a lot of information to be learned about sea moss. Right now, we've yet to find a source that states all of the 92 different minerals that are found there. But it includes and isn't limited to the different ypes of minerals that are listed here, the benefits of this, and what it can do.

And as you can see from this list, sea moss is very important not just for the health of he body, but for a lot of the processes on different levels, and a lot of people can benefit rom this too. There's a lot of nutrients to be had in this, a lot which are ideal for your body, so you should definitely consider having sea moss whenever you can.

Chapter 4

The Benefits of Sea Moss

So What are the Benefits of Sea Moss?

Well, there are a lot. Besides the immune benefits of sea moss, there is a lot. It can actually help on many different parts of the body, and there are a lot of benefits to be had. In this chapter, we'll go over some of the major benefits of sea moss, not just on the level of what it can do for the body, but also some of the other way's sea moss can help improve your life.

Hair, Nail, and Skin Benefits of Sea Moss

For starters, let's talk about what sea moss can do for the skin, hair and nails.

And it is a lot.

Remember what we said in the previous chapter, how it contains collagen. Well the collagen levels in sea moss are definitely not something to be underestimated, and they contribute to the health of skin, hair and nails of your body, so it's definitely a benefit for many of us.

But it's a natural antioxidant too, which means that toxins that normally sit there at the base and prevent healthy hair growth get eliminated, creating healthier, better hair. It also is an antimicrobial too, so you can also treat dandruff and inflammation as well, which is great for natural hair.

It also naturally conditions the hair. So for those with wavy hair, it actually is incredibly beneficial, and for natural hair that's 4c, it does detangle it. That's not to say it isn't good for other types of hair too, but for wavy and natural hair, it's great.

It also helps create shinier hair that's stronger. Due to the collagen that's within it, it can help with improving the overall look, creating more natural hair and preventing dullness too.

But what about in the skin? Well it's actually a powerhouse! Due to the antibacterial, antimicrobial, and antiviral properties, it actually balances out the biome of the skin, which can help reduce the oil production in the skin, and helps with making oily skin manageable. It also contains a ton of sulfur too, so it can help with balancing out the biome, and also can help with bacteria formation.

It also has some antibacterial effects too. Acne bacteria can be diminished with sea moss, and it can reduce acne severity. But not just that, it also contains sulfur, magnesium, calcium, and Vitamins A-K, which help with reducing the presence of wrinkles, helps with hydration, and protects from the elements.

Sea Moss and Weight Loss

Yes, sea moss can help you shed those pounds.

This is due to the iodine that's in the foods that's there. Since our bodies need this for thyroid hormones, it can help to properly balance out the thyroid gland. This is great for both brain and bone growth especially for younger people and for those who are pregnant.

However, you need to be careful with this, because too much iodine can cause an overabundance of thyroid hormones, which may cause an imbalanced thyroid. It is important that you don't use this as a sole weight loss supplement, and make sure that you don't have any possible risks for thyroid issues if you take this. With a thyroid supplement, you need to make sure that it's moderate at best.

However, more important than anything, sea moss is actually great for building lean muscles. It has 6 grams of protein for every 100 grams of sea moss, so there is a lot of protein there. However, it isn't just that either. It has something in there called taurine, which is important for not only burning fat, but also building muscle. It helps you burn fat rather than carbs when running, so if you take this before you hit the Stairmaster or going running, this can be a great way to help you build that muscle more than anything else.

Energy Galore

Sea moss contains something called iron in it, which of course, is really good for your energy levels. This is usually found in seafood, meat, and poultry as well. This has 9 mg of iron for every 100 grams, so it has about 9 times more than chicken.

You read that right, you can get more energy from sea moss than even chicken.

Low iron isn't good for you, since it can immediately sap your energy levels, so if you start to feel fatigued, that might be why.

The solution? Sea moss.

Sea moss gives you iron, which helps those red blood cells move the oxygen that's in your lungs to the cells, providing oxygen for them so they don't go into anaerobic respiration either.

This is a great addition for a lot of people, and there are some great ways to get sea moss. For example, adding it to smoothies is a good place to start, since it can give you a bunch of energy. This is also great for anemics too, since it can give them the iron they need to feel better.

Sea Moss and Mental Health

Sea moss has neuroactive characteristics which offer neuroprotective effects. This actually means that it can protect you from neurodegenerative disease.

Sea moss in particular can help slow down the growth of Parkinson's disease. Because of the potassium in the body, it can help with giving nutrients to the cells, improving the cognitive behavior and function. It is good for anxiety, depression, and even agitation and also other issues including fibromyalgia.

The B vitamins as well are great for the nervous system, and of course energy creation, and it can reduce signs of stress too.

Intimacy Benefits

If you take sea moss, it actually can help with your libido and sex drive. It can increase sex drive to higher levels.

This is due primarily to the zinc and other minerals within it, and libido increases through this. It also can help improve your self-esteem too, which is great to have before you start getting with your partner.

It is also great for women in particular, since having dryness down there can affect the intimacy. This can help with balancing out the pH of the area down there, and it can help provide lubrication. It also does help naturally promote the healthy growth of vaginal flora as well.

This is an effective solution in most cases, and also, it does help with reducing stress, which can be something great if you're feeling on edge as well.

Fertility Benefits

Some reports say sea moss can help with fertility, especially for those wishing to have a kid.

It is a good source of folate, but you should also be careful about that, and the iodine as well in the body.

The folic acid in there can also help with it. That's associated with fertility boosts and also improving your overall health. It also includes zinc, and other antioxidants, which are good for both.

Men should also take these too. That's because the minerals within this can help improve the quality and quantity of the sperm, improving your health, and improving the chances of this.

While it shouldn't be the only thing that you have, a sea moss smoothie may be a great addition to your pregnancy routine.

A Prebiotic?

In some studies, especially one that was published in the BMC Complementary Medicine and Therapies it was found that the sea moss consumed actually creates a prebiotic effect in some animals.

It can up your fatty acids within your colon, can help reduce bad gut bacteria, and help with the immune system.

Your gut is connected to your overall health, so this is something which can be good. In some cases, it also may stimulate digestion of nutrients and your metabolism.

While it isn't the only thing you should take, it may be beneficial to integrate this directly into your diet as well.

Thyroid Health and Sea Moss

Sea moss is great for thyroid health.

That again, is due to the iodine in this. It can help to naturally balance out the thyroid if it stops being active. The iodine in this starts to help stimulate the thyroid hormones in the body, which of course can stimulate production of such. This of course, helps keep the body properly regulated.

Your metabolism, your body temperature, and pretty much everything is based on the health of your thyroid, so if it starts to go out of whack, or you're at risk for gout, this can be a great thing. Sea moss has a lot of iodine though, so you should talk to your doctor before you try sea moss, since it could possibly affect the state of your thyroid, and may possibly overstimulate it too.

Digestive Health

Sea moss is actually great for optimizing the digestive system. It contains different minerals to help with balancing out the digestive tract. It also has a soothing agent which is good for the mucus membrane within your body. Due to the mucilaginous texture of Irish sea moss in particular, it can be great for a lot of people's digestive health, and can soothe a stomach.

It's great for stomach ulcers too.

This also can benefit the short-chain acids which are fatty in your colon, which can help with flushing out toxins.

It also can naturally get rid of bad bacteria in the gut too, balancing it out, which in turn helps with immunity too.

It also contains folate too, which is good for improving your DNA and other compounds too, and it is a great plant-based substitute for some dishes too.

Immunity and Fighting Colds

Sea moss is wonderful for your immune system because of the antioxidants in there. That means, it's anti-inflammatory so it will destroy free radicals, and aging too.

But more than that, it can fight off bacteria and viruses too, which can help with cold and flu symptoms.

This can be used directly with the onset of a cold if you're trying to prevent it from happening, and it helps you with recovering from the sickness too.

It also contains potassium chloride, which is great for inflammation and reducing the prospect of infection, and it has a great impact on your immune system. It's one of the best things to have for not just your gut, but for your immune system too, so it's a win if you take it regardless!

Other Benefits of Sea Moss

Sea moss can help with other things too.

It can help provide structure and support to our DNA, creating more red blood cells in the body, which helps oxygenate all of our organs.

They're also rich in minerals, and those are great for the body. It helps with improving mucous membranes as well, so if you have a cold or some decongestion, this can help with this.

It also is very rich in amino acids too, including sulfur, which can make the bones a lot stronger down the line.

It can help treat burns and eczema too, and it can offer treatment for rashes too.
It's also anti-diabetic, since it doesn't have any sugars or large amounts of carbs, and it can help with regulating blood glucose levels.

Overall, it's a wonderful way for you to get whatever you need. They contain minerals and vitamins that are vital for the body, can help with improving everything from your metabolism to even your mood, and it's perfect if you need that pick-me-up.

Chapter 5

What You Need to Know Before Buying Sea Moss

Preparation

How you prepare sea moss really depends on what you plan to do with it. Are you going to cook with it, use it as a gel, or add it to skincare items?

Well, no matter what, you need to do the following:

1. Take the sea moss and rinse it with some spring water, and check for debris and sand

2. Put it in water at room temperature for 4-24 hours at a time, rinsing every few hours

3. It will become a white, translucent color, and it will feel slippery and soft, with doubling in size

4. Drain the water and rinse them

5. Next, you can add spring water to this and put it in a blender.

6. Blend this until creamy and smooth

7. Put in a mason jar overnight to allow an hour of thickening

Once that's done, you can then use sea moss for various things, from smoothies to even skincare!

How Much Sea Moss Can I take?

Usually, a tablespoon or two is more than enough for you each day, but you can take up to ¼ cup. However, for those who have a thyroid condition please talk to your doctor. If you have a sea moss allergy or may suspect it, please consult your doctor too before taking it.

Side Effects of Sea Moss?

There may be some side effects of sea moss depending on whether or not you have thyroid conditions. If you have autoimmune thyroid issues such as Hashimoto's, this can cause issues such as hypothyroidism.

You also may put yourself at risk if you have too much iodine each day. But, it's also rare for you to have this happen.

There is also some risk with the different minerals in it. It does have a lot of aluminum, so it may not be healthy in the long term especially if you have heavy metals in the body.

Also, it may end up not being as effective in certain ways, since the FDA does not regulate this, so if you're buying from a third party seller, it may be risky.

Quality Degradation and Diseases Involving Sea Moss

Some species of sea moss can be prone to diseases and pests. There is one disease that affects sea moss which is called ice-ice, which can impact the moss, making it look frozen in a sense.

This can affect the salinity, the quality of this, and it may provide some bacteria a haven to flourish, which compromises the plant.

You don't want to get this, since it's basically like a woody pineapple, affecting the quality of the seaweed.

While rare, some third party sellers may give you this, and if you notice an icy look to the seaweed, that's a sign something may be wrong.

Packaging and Processing of Sea Moss

When you're buying this kind of seaweed, you should see if they have a clear photo of their batch of sea moss, and look to see if there is debris.

Check their packaging to make sure that they have air-tight bags, so it won't be subjected to the elements.

You should also look at the sediment of this, since it can mean the sea moss is susceptible to the debris that's on the surface, which contends with this.

Cultivation and Harvesting Considerations Involving Sea Moss

Finally, you want to make sure that they're grown and harvested effectively. Some seaweed farmers struggle with growing sea moss when the water is murky. If the water is clear, they can see the sediment there.

Sometimes, some of these plants are hurt by the sediment, and most cultivators won't even harvest that to process. When looking for sea moss, look for good farmers that won't risk their repute for a poor quality product.

You also should see a grade on the package of sea moss or from the retailer, which affects the price of this. Obviously, if you want a high quality sea moss product, you want a higher grade, and of course higher price.

Some farmers usually get only the product that works, and will abandon poor-quality products.

You may also want to consider the certifications as well that are present too. Usually, these companies have to go through a lot to get the right product, and any other relevant information.

You should make sure that they have certification that shows that they're compliant, and meet the criteria for what you want. Sea moss farming and processing is actually not that easy to get information out of farmers, so keep that in mind.

That's really what you need to know about sea moss, and important facts to consider as well.

Chapter 6

10 Delicious Smoothies that Use Sea Moss Gel

And here are 10 smoothies which use sea moss gel, including their nutritional facts as well.

Cacao Sea Moss Smoothie

Who doesn't love a fun and simple chocolate smoothie? This is pretty nice, and it tastes a bit frothy too due to the milk, and the vanilla that was added to this, and it comes with many health benefits, especially the Irish sea moss.

Ingredients:

- ☐ ½ ounce Irish sea moss
- ☐ A frozen banana
- ☐ 2-4 tablespoons cacao powder
- ☐ A pinch Himalayan pink salt
- ☐ A dash of cinnamon
- ☐ 4 cups almond milk
- ☐ 4-6 pitted medjool dates
- ☐ 1 tablespoon coconut oil
- ☐ ½ vanilla bean scraped
- ☐ A dash of nutmeg

Nutritional facts:

Calories: 100
Fat: 6 g
Sodium: 10 mg
Fiber: 3 g
Protein: 15 g
Carbohydrates: 3 g

Directions:

1. Take all ingredients and put them in a blender
2. Blend until made creamy! You can change up the thickness by adding more moss as well

Sea Moss Apple Smoothie

This is a simple sea moss smoothie perfect for those who love apples. It combines this into a wonderful, tantalizing and amazing apple taste that you won't be able to get enough of, and it also comes with some other health benefits, including properties of garlic, not normally seen in regular smoothies.

Ingredients:

- ☐ 2 cups apple juice
- ☐ 1 tablespoon ginger
- ☐ 1 dash garlic cloves
- ☐ 2 cups ice cubes
- ☐ 1 tablespoon sea moss gel
- ☐ 1 frozen banana
- ☐ 1 dash ground cinnamon

Nutritional facts:

Calories: 65
Fat: 1 g
Sodium: 7 mg
Protein: 10 g
Fiber: 3 g
Carbohydrates 5 g

Directions:

1. Take all of the ingredients, place in blender, blend until it's smooth
2. When ready, serve immediately to enjoy it!

Superfood Sea Moss Smoothie

This is a great smoothie because not only does it involve sea moss, but also some other amazing superfoods too. Sea moss is not your only superfood, and this low-calorie power smoothie is great for getting all of the nutritional elements that you're going for simply, and effectively as well.

Ingredients:

- ☐ 4 oz sea moss gel
- ☐ 1 ½ cups spring water
- ☐ ½ teaspoon ground cinnamon
- ☐ 2/5 tablespoons honey or agave
- ☐ 1 cup frozen soursop pulp
- ☐ 2 tablespoons minced ginger

☐ 1 teaspoon lemon juice, fresh

Nutritional facts:

Calories: 75
Fat: 2g
Sodium: 12 mg
Protein: 10 g
Fiber: 4 g
Carbohydrates: 3 g

Directions:

1. Take everything and put it in a blender
2. Add another cup of water if you want a smoother smoothie
3. Blend it all together until it's smoothed out
4. Drink it immediately!

Sea Moss Banana Smoothie

If you're a fan of bananas, especially those in your smoothies, this is a great one. It also has a rich, vanilla taste to it too, which is perfect for those who not only are looking for something that's a little bit healthy, but also a fun, sweet treat that you will definitely enjoy and love.

Ingredients:
☐ 2 frozen bananas
☐ ¼ cup organic hemp seeds
☐ ¾ teaspoon cinnamon
☐ 1 teaspoon vanilla
☐ 2-3 dates, pitted
☐ 3 tablespoons sea moss, prepared
☐ ¼ teaspoon nutmeg
☐ 3-5 black peppercorns
☐ 2 cups filtered water
☐ ½ jaggery
☐ 2 pinches cardamom
☐ 6-8 ice cubes
☐ Pinch of sea salt

Nutritional facts:

Calories: 125
Fat: 10g
Sodium: 30 mg
Protein: 15 g

Fiber: 7g
Carbohydrates: 9g

Directions:

1. Take everything and throw it in a blender, but add the water last so you have enough just for the blender contents
2. When you have everything in, pulse it, wait till it's blended, and then served
3. If it becomes too thick, you can add more water to improve the consistency
4. Serve!

Chocolate Raspberry Sea Moss Smoothie

Ingredients:

- ☐ ½ an avocado
- ☐ 1 ½ cups frozen raspberries
- ☐ 2 tablespoons raw cacao powder
- ☐ 1 ½ cups almond milk, or non-dairy milk
- ☐ Ice as needed
- ☐ 1 tablespoon flax seeds, ground
- ☐ 1 small cucumber
- ☐ ¼ cup sea moss gel
- ☐ 3 Medjool dates with the pits removed

Nutritional facts:

Calories: 332
Fat: 20 g
Sodium: 33mg
Protein: 25g
Fiber: 10g
Carbohydrates: 30g

Directions:

1. Take all of this and combine it together in a blender until it's smoothed out
2. You can add more almond milk to make it thicker, or add ice if you want a smoothie that's a bit thinner until the consistency is reached
3. This makes two smoothies, and they last up to a day in a mason jar that's airtight
4. You can add protein powder to these as well, and they're wonderful as a meal replacement

Pineapple Banana Smoothie

This is a simple tropical smoothie but having it will make you feel like you're at the beach, sipping away and having a wonderful time. It is a wonderful tropical treat, and with the addition of sea moss inside of it, it has the amazing effects of sea moss that you know and love, and ones that you will enjoy as well!

Ingredients:

- ☐ 1 cup strawberries
- ☐ 1 banana, frozen is best
- ☐ ½ cup Greek yogurt
- ☐ 1 tablespoons flaxseed or chia seeds
- ☐ ¼ tablespoon sea moss
- ☐ ½ cup pineapple
- ☐ 2 cups orange juice
- ☐ 1 cup of spinach, optional
- ☐ Ice for thickening

Nutritional facts:

Calories: 135
Fat: 10g
Sodium: 30mg
Protein: 20g
Fiber: 10g
Carbohydrates: 37g

Directions:

1. Make sure your bananas are frozen and your spinach is chopped up
2. Take all of those ingredients and throw them into a blender k
3. Blend until smooth, adding more ice as needed if you feel it needs to be thickened up a bit
4. Serve immediately

Sweet Cherry Smoothie

Who doesn't love a sweet and succulent smoothie? Well, you can have that, and the amazing taste of cherries in this simple smoothie. It has a lot of protein in it too, so it may be a great meal replacement if you want a simple, powerful smoothie that comes with some health benefits you may not normally get.

Ingredients:

- ☐ 2 cups frozen cherries
- ☐ 1 scoop protein powder
- ☐ Ice

- [ ] 1 cup almond milk
- [ ] ½ teaspoon sea moss
- [ ] 1 banana, frozen
- [ ] Coconut flakes and almond butter for topping

Nutritional facts:

Calories: 157
Fat: 10g
Sodium: 15mg
Protein: 30g
Fiber: 6g
Carbohydrates: 35g

Directions:

1. Take all of the ingredients and put them in the blender
2. With the almond milk, you can add more if you want a thicker smoothie.
3. Blend it until it's properly mixed
4. Top with unsweetened flakes, or the almond butter

Greens and Sea Moss Smoothie

Getting greens has never been easier. With this sea moss smoothie, all of those greens that you love will definitely be in this. It's full of rich antioxidants, and vitamins and minerals that your body needs. It's quite rewarding, and it's a great addition to your sea moss smoothie repertoire, and you definitely shouldn't discount this either.

Ingredients:

- [ ] 2 cup pineapple, frozen or otherwise
- [ ] ½ cup grapes
- [ ] 1 banana
- [ ] ½ tablespoon sea moss
- [ ] 2 cups spinach, broken up
- [ ] 2 cups orange juice
- [ ] A banana
- [ ] Some ice

Nutritional facts:

Calories: 129
Fat: 2g
Sodium: 8mg
Protein: 25g
Fiber: 10g

Carbohydrates: 15g

Directions:

1. Take all of the ingredients and put them in a blender
2. Add ice if you want a thicker smoothie
3. Pulsate this until properly blended
4. Serve it immediately

Chocolate Power Smoothie

Chocolate AND protein? It's all there in this simple, powerful smoothie. It's packed with a lot of protein, and enough fat to keep you satisfied and a great mal replacement in many cases. It's a great one to have if you're looking for a sea moss recipe that you can enjoy, and one that's simple enough for anyone to use.

Ingredients:

- ☐ 1 cup coconut milk
- ☐ ½ cup blueberries
- ☐ A banana
- ☐ Some ice
- ☐ 2 tablespoons sea moss.
- ☐ A scoop of chocolate protein powder
- ☐ A cup of spinach
- ☐ A tablespoon of almond butter

Nutritional Information:

Calories: 220
Fat: 20g
Sodium: 5mg
Protein: 33g
Fiber: 9g
Carbohydrates: 30g

Directions:

1. With the protein powder, you can use your favorite one, or even a low-calorie alternative
2. Mix them together, using more milk or ice to improve the consistency of the smoothie
3. When combined, pour into a cup and serve
4. This should be drank immediately

Youthful Glow Sea Moss Smoothie

This is a great smoothie that not only uses sea moss in order to help you have healthier skin and hair, but also some other important elements that will help you keep a nice, youthful glow to your hair, skin, and body as well. It comes with some amazing fruits that will definitely leave your palate begging for more, and more and more of a desire for some amazing smoothie options.

Ingredients:

- [ ] 2 handfuls of kale or power greens
- [ ] 2 cups apple juice, organic
- [ ] ½ squeezed lemon or use juice from a full lemon
- [ ] 2 handfuls of baby spinach
- [ ] ½ a cucumber
- [ ] A banana
- [ ] Some ice
- [ ] A teaspoon of fresh and grated ginger
- [ ] 4 oz of sea moss gel

Nutritional Facts:

Calories: 157
Fat: 1g
Sodium: 3mg
Protein: 10g
Fiber: 8g
Carbohydrates: 16g

Directions:

1. Make sure to properly prepare the power greens and kale, cutting it off the stems as needed
2. Make sure to squeeze the lemon juice out of this and then put it in there
3. Grate the ginger if not done already
4. Take everything and put it all into a blender
5. Blend this until smooth, adding some water into it to help make it easier to drink
6. Serve it immediately!

And there you have it, 10 amazing sea moss smoothies that you will definitely not be able to get enough of. They're simple, yet effective, and are great if you're looking for sea moss recipes that you definitely can benefit from, and some amazing benefits that are sitting there just waiting for you too.

Conclusion

Sea moss is powerful. In fact, it's something that ancient cultures have been using for years. With the variety of different properties that are in place, it's no wonder that people enjoy the mouth-watering, refreshing taste of sea moss smoothies.

You can also use this in different ways too. It isn't just a smoothie, but you can use this in your hair, skin, and even with cooking in your favorite dishes. And the properties are all there.

This is a superfood that some people don't even know about, and the miraculous properties that come along with this definitely are worth mentioning. There are so many good things for you to get out of sea moss, and a lot of people do benefit immensely from these amazing characteristics that sea moss has to offer.

And you can get them too. There are so many properties of sea moss out there just waiting to be achieved, and many people don't realize that the full benefits of this are definitely interesting, and innovative too.

The next step for you to take of course, is to use sea moss in a recipe, or use it how you want. Go online, and take some time to look for the proper retailer to work with. Remember, you want a high-quality recipe that will benefit you, and something that has a variety of different properties that are good for you. If you find it's packaged in great ways, then great! You can from there, choose to of course, buy it, and work from there.

You can use sea moss in different ways, and while it may work differently for everyone, using it as a supplement, and as a superfood is really good.

However, if you are someone who has a thyroid condition, it may be best for you to talk to your doctor before starting this, and make sure that you aren't harming yourself by taking sea moss.

Thank You

Thank you for buying my book and I hope you enjoyed it. If you found any value in this book I would really appreciate it if you'd take a minute to post a review on Amazon about this book. I check all my reviews and love to get feedback.

This is the real reward for me knowing that I'm helping others. If you know anyone who may enjoy this book, please share the message and gift it to them.

Other Books By Author

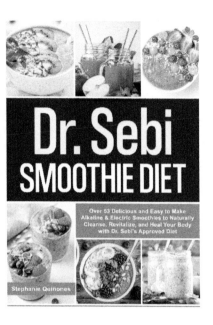

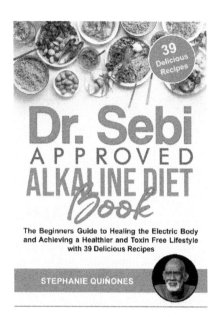

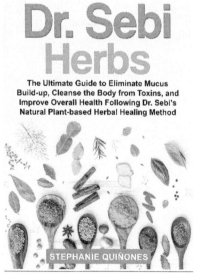

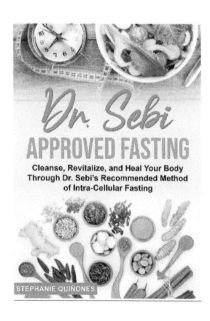

About Author

My name is Stephanie Quiñones, an entrepreneur living in the United States who loves sharing knowledge and helping others on the topic of weight-loss, healthy eating, anti-aging, and improving love life.

I'm a very passionate person who will go the extra mile and over-delivers to inspire others to lose weight, be healthy, and to achieve the sexy body they desire.

Stephanie's words of wisdom:

"I believe that knowledge is power. Everyone should improve themselves and/or business, no matter what stage in life they're in. Whether it's to develop a better mindset or to increase profits. Moving forward is key."

Printed in Great Britain
by Amazon

25660929R00030